# Obesity Relevant Pharmacology Vignettes

# &

# Multiple Choice Questions



**Muhammad Asad MD**

# Editor

Muhammad Asad MD, FACS, FASMBS

Diplomate American Board of Obesity Medicine

Bariatric and Minimally Invasive Surgeon

# Preface

Obesity is still a growing problem and a major health concern in USA and many parts of the world. A significant number of healthcare providers are showing special interest in learning about this complex disease. This book is put together to focus on pharmacological aspects. There is paucity of literature regarding this very aspect. Pace of introduction of new drugs in managing obesity is very slow. Some medications have been pulled from market due to potential risks. Clear evidence-based guidelines are lacking regarding dosing for many commonly used medications. Failure to assess correct dosing may not only compromise desired therapeutic effects but also risks toxicity in some situations.

An effort is made in this book to discuss weight loss medications and to cover commonly used medications in other related clinical scenarios. Cues are taken from day-to-day real life clinical problems to formulate vignettes and multiple-choice questions.

This book will be a resource for those preparing for the obesity certification examination. This will also be a good problem-based learning tool for the healthcare professionals already in practice.

Feedback from the readers is very valuable. It helps steer the direction of work and improvement efforts.

I feel this book will be a valuable contribution to the existing literature. Questions derived from actual clinical problems will help the readers fill gaps in understanding and improve knowledge to become better clinicians.

Finally, I would like to thank all my colleagues especially Dr. Tawsufe Majid and Dr. Saima Ashraf who helped in formulating this manuscript.

Muhammad Asad FACS, FASMBS
Diplomate American Board of Obesity Medicine

# Disclaimer



Although every possible precaution has been made to ensure the accuracy of the information contained in this book, the author and publisher assume no responsibility for any errors or omissions. No liability is assumed for damages that may result from the use of information contained in this publication.

**Question 1**

Which of the following statements is correct about the use of phentermine in the management of obesity?

a. Phentermine has been in clinical use since 1959 and carries a very significant addicting potential.

b. FDA approved phentermine for long-term use up to 36 weeks

c. BMI thresholds are best tools to aid in decision making when prescribing phentermine and the patients should be seen at least every six months.

d. Phentermine belongs to a group of substituted phenethylamines

e. Phentermine does not produce false positive urine drug screen tests

The correct answer is "d."

Phentermine is a controlled medicine and belongs to schedule IV category. It requires a prescription. It does not carry significant addiction potential. FDA has approved it for short-term use. A consensus does not exist about how frequently patients should be followed. Six months seems to be a too long time for follow-up. False positive drug screen tests may occur for amphetamine or methamphetamine while taking phentermine. This may require specific tests to differentiate.

Hendricks, E. J., Rothman, R. B., & Greenway, F. L. (2009). How Physician Obesity Specialists Use Drugs to Treat Obesity. Obesity, 17(9), 1730-1735. doi:10.1038/oby.2009.69

https://www.verywellmind.com/how-long-does-adipex-stay-in-your-system-80217

**Question 2**

Which of the following statements is correct regarding the pharmacology of phentermine?

a. Phentermine base and phentermine hydrochloride have the same potency

b. Phentermine has a half-life of 4 hours.

c. Phentermine is known to have teratogenic effects during pregnancy

d. Titration of the dose of phentermine is not needed

e. Adult obese patients with ADHD may require higher doses of phentermine

The correct answer is "e."

The half-life of phentermine hydrochloride is 7 to 20 hours. Titration of phentermine dose is generally required. It is the observation by some physicians that patients with a diagnosis of ADHD need higher doses of phentermine. There are no teratogenic effects ascribed to phentermine. This drug is not recommended in pregnancy since FDA recommendations in 1979.

Steelman, G. M., & Westman, E. C. Pharmacotherapy. In: Steelman, G. M., & Westman, E. C. (Eds.) Obesity: evaluation and treatment essentials, 2nd Edition. Boca Raton: CRC Press, Taylor & Francis Group Press; 2016, pp.141-145

## Question 3

A 28-year-old patient with current symptoms of ADHD and chronic diarrhea is started on phentermine. The patient is currently not on any other stimulants. Please select the correct statement.

a. A decreased heart rate is expected

b. Appetite is likely to increase

c. Diarrhea may improve

d. Symptoms of ADHD will increase

e. Intestinal motility will increase

The correct answer is "c."

The adrenergic effect may lead to an increase in heart rate, decrease in appetite, improvement of diarrhea and ADHD symptoms. Intestinal activity may decrease.

## Question 4

A 35-year-old patient with morbid obesity is prescribed phentermine. She experienced significant insomnia several months after starting the medication. A diagnosis of late-onset insomnia was made. Which of the following statements is <u>not</u> correct regarding managing her symptom?

a. Phentermine dose may be decreased

b. Phentermine may need to be stopped

c. Pindolol may help

d. Benzodiazepines are preferred for this kind of insomnia

e. Trazodone may be tried

The correct answer is "d."

Late-onset insomnia occurs in less than 1 in 1000 patients. It sometimes responds to melatonin, pindolol or trazodone. Benzodiazepines are generally not recommended for this type of insomnia. Early onset insomnia usually responds to pindolol at bedtime.

**Question 5**

A 40-year-old patient with a BMI of 37 is prescribed phentermine. She experiences constipation, lightheadedness, difficulty in micturition and dry mouth. Some of these effects can be explained based on which of the following mechanisms?

a. Cholinergic effects
b. Adrenergic effects
c. Anticholinergic effects
d. Antiadrenergic effects
e. Antidopaminergic effects

The correct answer is "c."

The side effects mentioned above are anticholinergic in nature.

**Question 6**

Which of the following statements is correct about Diethylpropion?

a. Its half-life is similar to phentermine
b. It may be a useful alternate drug for weight loss for people experiencing insomnia with phentermine
c. Its use is considered safe during pregnancy
d. Its use is safe for children below 16 years
e. Diethylpropion cannot be combined with other weight loss medications.

The correct answer is "b."

This medicine has a half-life of 4 to 6 hours. It has been used in patients with the problem of insomnia. This drug is not recommended for pediatric patients and during pregnancy since FDA assigned it category B in 1979. This medicine has been used in combinations with other weight loss drugs.

Cercato, C., Roizenblatt, V. A., Leança, C. C., Segal, A., Filho, A. P., Mancini, M. C., & Halpern, A. (2009). A randomized, double-blind placebo-controlled study of the long-term efficacy and safety of diethylpropion in the treatment of obese subjects. International Journal of Obesity, 33(8), 857-865. doi:10.1038/ijo.2009.124

**Question 7**

Orlistat has been used in the treatment of obesity. Select the correct statement.

a. Orlistat has been proven to be very successful in clinical practice
b. Its mechanism of action is about inhibition of intestinal lipase to prevent absorption of fat.
c. It can produce oily diarrhea and foul-smelling flatus
d. Its use is not considered safe for children below 16 years
e. b and c are correct

The correct answer is "e."

Due to the side effects, this medicine has not been very successful in clinical practice. It is considered safe for use in the pediatric age group under 16.

**Question 8**

A 28-year-old morbidly obese female is interested in starting Phentermine and Topiramate combination for weight loss. She is normotensive. She has history of renal stones. Which of the following statements is correct about the use of this combination?

a. She needs counseling about risks of birth defects involving craniofacial deformities.
b. She can nurse her baby as these medicines are not excreted in milk.

c. Her chances of having renal stones in future are not increased

d. She may experience dry mouth, and this effect can be due to both Topiramate and phentermine

e. a and d are correct

The correct answer is "e."

Birth defects especially cleft lip and palate may be associated with Topamax use. Safety of these drugs in nursing mothers has not been established. There is some risk of renal stones with use of Topamax. A likely reason for this may be the metabolic acidosis produced by Topamax. Dry mouth can be a troublesome side effect of this combination. Some of the other side effects include paresthesia, oligohydrosis, and hyperkalemia. Topiramate inhibits carbonic anhydrase. Zonisamide (another antiepileptic) has also been reported to cause weight loss.

**Question 9**

Lorcaserin (Belviq®) have been pulled out of market due to which of the following reasons?

a. Risk of GI tumors

b. Risk of Serotonin syndrome

c. Risk of development of cardiac murmurs

d. Addiction risks

e. All the above statements are correct.

The correct answer is "a."

This medication was recalled from the marked due to risks of development of various tumors especially involving gastrointestinal system, lung, and breast.

**Question 10**

A 55-year morbidly obese patient with BMI 45 is interested in starting Bupropion/naltrexone combination for weight loss. She has degenerative spine disease and bulging discs. She uses ibuprofen for pain control. Please select the correct statement about the use of this combination.

a. This medication combination is not contraindicated due to concurrent use of NSAIDs.

b. The incremental dose is needed in the first few weeks to avoid some of the side effects

c. Side effect of nausea is generally due to naltrexone component

d. This drug does not fall in the category of controlled substances as classified by DEA

e. All the above statements are correct

The correct answer is "e."

Bupropion is an antidepressant and naltrexone is an opioid receptor antagonist. This combination cannot be used if patient is taking narcotic medications. However, it can be used if NSAIDs are prescribed for pain control. An incremental dose of the combination is recommended to avoid some of the side effects.

Nausea occurs due to naltrexone component. This drug is not classified as a controlled medicine.

Greenway, F. L., Dunayevich, E., Tollefson, G., Erickson, J., Guttadauria, M., Fujioka, K., & Cowley, M. A. (2009). Comparison of Combined Bupropion and Naltrexone Therapy for Obesity with Monotherapy and Placebo. The Journal of Clinical Endocrinology & Metabolism, 94(12), 4898-4906. doi:10.1210/jc.2009-1350

**Question 11**

Topiramate has been used in combination with phentermine or alone in obesity management for many years. Which of the following statements is correct about the use of this medication?

a. This medication is found to be useful in controlling binge eating and weight gain due to antidepressant medication use.

b. FDA has not approved this medication for weight loss, so its use for this condition is regarded as "Off-label." Patients need to be counseled about this.

c. Neurologic symptoms are due to its weak inhibition of carbonic anhydrase activity

d. Acute closed-angle Glaucoma is an idiosyncratic reaction of topiramate and should be urgently addressed with appropriate referral and stopping the medication.

e. All the above statements are correct

The correct answer is "e."

Topiramate is a commonly used off-label drug for weight loss. It is found to be useful for controlling hunger symptoms. It helps reduce craving for carbohydrates and sweets. Beneficial effects are observed in disorders like binge eating and drug-induced weight gain after use of antidepressants. Acute closed angle glaucoma can precipitate with topiramate use in patients with narrow angles. The condition requires emergent attention. It can result in blindness if not addressed promptly.

Atrup A, Caterrson I, Zelissen P, Guy-Grand B, Carruba M, Levy B, et al. (2004). Topiramate long-term maintenance of weight loss induced by a low-calorie diet in obese subjects Obes Res 12,1658-1669

**Question 12**

Which of the following statements is correct about Liraglutide?

a. It is a GLP-1 receptor agonist

b. It is a GLP-1 receptor antagonist

c. It decreases insulin release

d. It increases glucagon release

e. It increases food intake and promotes weight gain

The correct answer is "a."

Liraglutide is a long-acting GLP-1 analog. This activates the GLP-1 receptor in the pancreatic islet cells. It increases insulin release and lowers glucagon secretion. This drug reduces food intake and promotes weight loss. This may also increase the risk of medullary thyroid neoplasm and pancreatitis.

Gorgojo-Martínez, J. J., Feo-Ortega, G., & Serrano-Moreno, C. (2016). Effectiveness and tolerability of liraglutide in patients with type 2 diabetes mellitus and obesity after bariatric surgery. Surgery for Obesity and Related Diseases, 12(10), 1856-1863. doi: 10.1016/j.soard.2016.02.013

**Question 13**

Which of the following statements is correct about pharmacological effects of Liraglutide?

a. It increases gastric emptying
b. It raises blood sugar
c. It decreases satiety
d. It decreases gastric emptying
e. It does not affect gastric emptying

The correct answer is "d."

Liraglutide is a GLP -1 agonist. It decreases gastric emptying time, reduces hunger, decreases caloric intake and blood sugar. These effects promote weight loss.

Niswender, K., Pi-Sunyer, X., Buse, J., Jensen, K. H., Toft, A. D., Russell-Jones, D., & Zinman, B. (2012). Weight change with liraglutide and comparator therapies: an analysis of seven phase 3 trials from the liraglutide diabetes development programme. Diabetes, Obesity and Metabolism, 15(1), 42-54. doi:10.1111/j.1463-1326.2012. 01673.x

## Question 14

A 39-year-old woman with BMI of 37, is seen in a Bariatric office. She describes premenstrual craving for chocolates, sugars, and carbohydrates. She has gained 20 pounds in the last three months. Her fat distribution is predominantly in pelvic area and thighs. Some edema of legs is noted as well. She has several high blood pressure readings, and family doctor is considering starting some antihypertensive medication. Appropriate nutritional counseling was done. Which of the following medications can be a <u>cost-effective</u> and useful option for her to reduce symptoms of food craving in addition to help control blood pressure and edema?

a. Spironolactone hydrochlorothiazide combination
b. Metoprolol
c. Hydralazine
d. Nafidipine
e. Captopril.

The correct answer is "a"

Some experienced authors have cited spironolactone /hydrochlorothiazide combination (25 mg dose for each) may be helpful in preventing some of the premenstrual symptoms of craving for sweets and carbohydrates in addition to treating high blood pressure and edema. This scenario highlights the importance of keeping patient's overall clinical picture in mind as multiple conditions can be addressed with a medication or a combination. Edema is common in obese patients. Clinicians need to differentiate edema from lipedema. The latter condition may respond to physical therapy and compression dressings. It may also need surgical intervention.

Steelman, G. M., & Westman, E. C. Pharmacotherapy. In: Steelman, G. M., & Westman, E. C. (Eds.) Obesity: evaluation and treatment essentials, 2nd Edition. Boca Raton: CRC Press, Taylor & Francis Group Press; 2016, pp.157

**Question 15**

A 37-year-old woman with BMI of 31 is prescribed liraglutide (Saxenda®) *. She is also known to have DM 2. A few months later she presents with severe upper abdominal pain along with nausea and vomiting. She has a white cell count of 14.3. Blood sugar is 280mg /dl, liver functions are normal, and urine analysis is in the normal range. Her blood sugars have not been very well controlled in the last few months. Which of the following statements is correct regarding her clinical condition?

a. GERD (gastroesophageal reflux disease) is a more likely diagnosis
b. Colitis is a common side effect of liraglutide
c. A CT scan of the abdomen may show stranding in retrogastric and duodenal C area
d. Ultrasound of the abdomen may not be very helpful
e. None of the above statements is true

The correct answer is "c."

Please see explanation with Question 16

*Saxenda® is a registered trademark of Novo Nordisk A/S

## Question 16

Patient in the above question was discharged later when her additional workup was found to be negative. She follows with her family doctor a few days later. She is considered for starting some additional medication to control diabetes. Which of the following statements is correct?

a. Insulin and liraglutide combination can be an option

b. Liraglutide dose should not be increased to have better control of diabetes

c. Liraglutide is not very cost effective for most patients

d. It is only available as an injection

e. All above statements are correct

The correct answer is "e."

Statements “a” to “d” are correct. Patients on Liraglutide carry an increased risk of developing pancreatitis and gallstones. Any acute upper abdominal pain needs evaluation with these diagnoses in mind. A CT scan study may show changes related to pancreatitis with stranding. Sonogram of the gallbladder may show stones or sludge.

Need Help Taking Off Excess Weight and Keeping It Off? (n.d.). Retrieved January 02, 2018, from https://www.saxenda.com/

**Question 17**

A 30-year-old morbidly obese male was diagnosed with HIV infection. Antiretroviral therapy was started with zidovudine. He is given handouts and links to the information about side effects of HIV medications. At his next family doctor's office visit, he asks several questions from his provider. Please select the correct statement.

a. He has decreased risk of hyperglycemia

b. He is less likely to have dyslipidemia

c. His visceral fat is likely to increase

d. He is less likely to develop lipodystrophy

e. Increased subcutaneous adiposity

The correct answer is "c."

Older HIV medications have led to lipodystrophy in many patients. Newer medications do not have this side effect.

“Factsheet Lipodystrophy.” HIV & AIDS Information, www.aidsmap.com/Lipodystrophy/page/1045065/.

**Question 18**

A 27-year-old morbidly obese female is diagnosed with polycystic ovarian syndrome (PCOS) and insulin resistance. Her liver functions are abnormal. Lab work show AST and ALT both raised by 30% from base values. She takes tricyclic antidepressants regularly. She is recently found to be HIV positive and considering antiretroviral therapy. She has recently joined a weight loss program. While taking history, it is also found that her father had colon cancer at the age of 45 and mother developed breast cancer at the age of 39 years. Her lab work shows slightly raised insulin levels. Which of the following medications may be a useful choice for her considering her existing list of multiple diagnoses and risk factors?

a. Phentermine
b. Sucralfate
c. Metformin
d. Naltrexone/bupropion combination
e. Topiramate

The correct answer is "c."

Metformin is considered useful for insulin resistance, fatty liver, and PCOS. It may be helpful in preventing some of the weight-related complications with use of anti retroviral medications. and some antidepressants. Another potential benefit exists in colon cancer prevention.

Johnson, N P. "Metformin Use in Women with Polycystic Ovary Syndrome." Annals of Translational Medicine., U.S. National Library of Medicine, June 2014, www.ncbi.nlm.nih.gov/pubmed/25333031.

**Question 19**

A 32-year-old morbidly obese female is followed in a bariatric program. She carries a BMI of 49. She has several stressors in life, and the recent loss of her mother has made her very depressed. She sees a counselor. A consideration is made by her family physician to start some antidepressant. Please select the medication which can be relatively weight neutral.

a. Imipramine

b. Paroxetine

c. Fluoxetine

d. Amitriptyline

e. Doxepin

The correct answer is "c."

Fluoxetine seems to be a better choice among the stated medications due to less weight gaining potential.

Hasnain, Mehrul, et al. “Weight Gain and Glucose Dysregulation with Second-Generation Antipsychotics and Antidepressants: A Review for Primary Care Physicians.” Postgraduate Medicine, vol. 124, no. 4, 2012, pp. 154–167., doi:10.3810/pgm.2012.07.2577.

**Question 20**

A 40-year-old male with BMI 37 follows a weight loss program. He has a history of depression for many years. Lately due to loss of job, depression has become worse. He smokes a pack daily for the last eight years. Discussion between the counselor, bariatrician and family doctor in the multidisciplinary meeting takes place.

Currently, he is on doxepin. Concerns are raised about the weight gaining potential of the medication. Reasonable choice for his symptoms of depression could be which one of the following medications?

a. Imipramine
b. Paroxetine
c. Bupropion
d. Amitriptyline
e. Doxepin

The correct answer is "c."

Bupropion seems to be a reasonable choice for him. It may be beneficial for control of depression symptoms along with help in quitting smoking. It may also help losing weight. Bupropion in combination with naltrexone is an approved weight loss medication.

## Question 21

A 30-year-old female with BMI 33 underwent sleeve gastrectomy procedure a couple of years ago. She has also undergone cholecystectomy and tubal ligation. She has lost 55 pounds of weight since surgery. She has started gaining weight for the last few months. She craves for chips and crackers in the evenings. She had severe anxiety and had developed panic attacks a few times in the recent months. She also has a history of migraines. Currently, she gets severe headaches which are affecting her quality of life. She follows a neurologist. Which of the following medications may help improve her symptoms?

a. Phentermine

b. Paroxetine

c. Bupropion

d. Topiramate

e. Bupropion and naltrexone combination

The correct answer is "d."

Here topiramate may be a better choice. It may address her issues of headaches and help improve cravings for starches. Phentermine should be avoided in her case due to anxiety and panic attacks. Use of Topamax for weight loss remains off-label. Any female with childbearing potential needs to be educated about pregnancy related risks with its use.

**Question 22**

Please select the medication which has the most potential of weight gain.

a. Clozapine

b. Trazodone

c. Benzodiazepines

d. Amisulpride

e. Melatonin

The correct answer is "a."

In this list of sedatives, clozapine has the most potential of weight gain.

**Question 23**

A 34-year-old lady is seeking help to lose weight in a weight loss program. Her medical reconciliation reveals methylphenidate (Ritalin®) prescribed for ADHD. She also takes medications for hypertension. Her blood pressure fluctuates. She has anxiety issues at times. She is given various options. She is interested in starting phentermine/topiramate combination to help control cravings for food. Please select the correct statement.

a. Phentermine and methylphenidate have very similar potential of producing dependence
b. Both medicines can be used safely together
c. Methylphenidate and phentermine should be avoided together as her blood pressure control may be affected
d. The patient may see more anxiety issues due to the stimulant nature of both medications if used simultaneously
e. "c" and "d" are correct

The correct answer is "e."

Phentermine is schedule IV, and methylphenidate is schedule II drug. Later has more potential for dependence. Concurrent use in her case should be avoided for reasons of stimulant nature and potential effect on her blood pressure.

Ritalin® is a registered trademark of Novartis Pharmaceuticals

## Question 24

Topiramate /phentermine combination is started for a morbidly obese patient to help control cravings for sweets and carbs. One week after starting the treatment she felt blurry vision and discomfort in eyes. She calls her physician's office. The provider suspects development of acute glaucoma. An emergency referral is arranged to see an ophthalmologist. Please select the correct statement about her clinical condition.

a. Her glaucoma is likely to be an open angle glaucoma
b. Drainage channels for aqueous humor in trabecular meshwork between iris and cornea are blocked
c. A defect in the ciliary body due to edema and displacement leading to closing the angle between iris and cornea is a likely reason
d. Alkaline phosphatase is a key enzyme in controlling the aqueous humor production
e. Topiramate increase carbonic anhydrase production

The correct answer is "c."

Acute narrow-angle glaucoma is reported as a complication with use of some of the weight loss medications including topiramate. It requires urgent evaluation and treatment. Blindness may result if a delay in treatment occurs. Topiramate is a weak inhibitor of carbonic anhydrase. This enzyme is involved in aqueous humor production.

## Question 25

A 52-year-old female is noted to have gained 20 pounds at her annual physical with her primary care physician. She has several medical problems. She has a long of list of medications. Some of the medications were started in the past year. At medical reconciliation, she is found to be taking metoprolol for hypertension, glipizide /metformin for diabetes, Gabapentin for chronic pain issues. She has started taking bupropion for depression a few months back. Please select the correct statement.

a. Both Metoprolol and bupropion can cause weight gain

b. Both Metformin and Gabapentin can cause weight gain

c. Both Glipizide and bupropion can cause weight gain

d. Both Metformin and bupropion can cause weight gain

e. Both Metformin and metoprolol can cause weight gain

f. Both Metoprolol and glipizide can cause weight gain

The correct answer is "f."

Metoprolol, glipizide, gabapentin can cause weight gain.

**Question 26**

Which of the following weight loss medication should not be used in patients with suicidal ideations?

a. Phentermine topiramate combination
b. Orlistat
c. Naltrexone HCL and bupropion combination

d. Liraglutide
e. None of the above medications is associated with suicidal ideation
f. Options a, c, and d

The correct answer is "f."

Phentermine topiramate combination, naltrexone bupropion combination and liraglutide should be avoided in patient with suicidal ideations.

https://www.drugs.com/disease-interactions/liraglutide,victoza.html

https://www.rxlist.com/contrave-drug.htm#warnings

**Question 27**

A 45-year-old female with BMI of 37 is started on Topiramate (off label) to help control cravings for sweets and carbohydrates. As part of follow up, a panel of labs is requested after a couple of months of use. Which of the following metabolic side effects is anticipated?

a. Metabolic acidosis
b. Metabolic alkalosis
c. Respiratory acidosis
d. Respiratory alkalosis

Correct answer is “a.”

Topiramate inhibits carbonic anhydrase, and it may lead to renal bicarbonate loss and development of metabolic acidosis.

**Questions 28**

Fatty liver disease management can be challenging. Please select the correct statement.

a. GLP1 agonists have an indirect beneficial effect on fatty liver by causing weight loss
b. Pioglitazone can help prevent the progression of fibrosis in fatty liver disease
c. Pioglitazone can precipitate CHF
d. 10 percent weight loss may improve NASH by 80%
e. All above statements are correct.

Correct answer is "e."

Pioglitazone belongs to thiazolidinedione class. It improves the sensitivity of insulin. Its side effects include bladder carcinoma, hypoglycemia, CHF, and osteoporosis. Contraindications include pregnancy and breast feeding.

**Question 29**

Glomerular filtration rate remains important in calculating doses of many pharmacological agents. Which of the following statements is correct about the estimated glomerular filtration rate in patients after bariatric surgery?

a. In post-bariatric surgery cases, estimated glomerular filtration rate (GFR) remains as one of most reliable methods of renal function assessment.

b. Estimated GFR does not depend on creatinine

c. Estimated GFR is likely to decrease in post-bariatric patients due to loss of muscle mass

d. Estimated GFR does not take into account the surface area of the patient

e. In post-bariatric surgery patients, estimated GFR may increase without real improvement of renal function

The correct answer is "e."

This interesting fact is derived from several observations. After bariatric surgery patients lose some muscle mass. GFR data tables are obtained from patients who are not obese and decreased body surface area after losing weight is not adjusted in GFR calculations. This issue may lead to incorrect estimations of GFR. Some of the equations used in the assessment of GFR include CKD-EPI, MDRD, and Cockcroft-Gault. The later one incorporates lean body mass adjustments.

Editorial Board. (2016). Surgery for Obesity and Related Diseases, 12(1), I-Ii. doi:10.1016/s1550-7289(15)01029-1

**Question 30**

Several medications are known to affect lipid and carbohydrate metabolism. Which of the following medications may lead to hyperglycemia, lipid disorder, decreased subcutaneous fat and more visceral fat accumulation?

a. Loop diuretics

b. Proton pump inhibitors

c. Antiretroviral therapy

d. Cephalosporins

e. Chronic coumadin use

The correct answer is "c."

Antiretroviral therapy is noted to have stated side effects. Metformin may help in preventing some of these effects.

**Question 31**

In evaluating an obese patient, it may be useful to have an assessment of fat-free mass and lean body mass. These calculations remain important in determining doses of some medications and nutritional goals. Please select the correct statement.

a. Lean body mass is total body mass minus fatty tissues. In a nonobese person it is generally 75% of total body mass.
b. Fat-free mass is total body mass minus total body fat.
c. Lean body mass differs from the fat free mass by approximately 5%
d. Fat-free mass can be measured with techniques like dual-energy x-ray absorptiometry (DXA) scan or bioelectrical impedance (BIA)
e. All the above statements are correct.

The correct answer is "e."

Fat-free mass is the sum of water, minerals, protein, and glycogen of body. On the other hand, lean body mass is the sum of water, mineral, protein, glycogen, fat in organs, bone marrow, and CNS.

**Question 32**

A 37-year-old lady had biliopancreatic diversion procedure with duodenal switch for super morbid obesity, eight years ago. She is seen in her family doctor's office for annual physical examination. She is complaining of bruises and heavy periods. She takes over the counter vitamins. Which of the following statements is correct about her clinical condition?

a. One of the group B water-soluble vitamin deficiencies could be a probable cause
b. Fat soluble vitamin deficiencies are infrequently seen
c. Vitamin E deficiency is likely reasons for her symptoms.
d. Vitamin K deficiency is seen in more than 50 % of patients with biliopancreatic diversion.
e. Vitamin K supplements are not helpful

The correct answer is "d."

Biliopancreatic diversion has a high metabolic impact due to significant malabsorption. Patients are vulnerable to develop multiple nutritional deficiencies. Fat-soluble vitamins need special attention. Fat soluble vitamin are A, D, E and K.

Fujioka, K., Dibaise, J. K., & Martindale, R. G. (2011). Nutrition and Metabolic Complications After Bariatric Surgery and Their Treatment. Journal of Parenteral and Enteral Nutrition, 35(5_suppl). doi:10.1177/0148607111413600

## Question 33

A 45-year-old lady presents to the bariatric office. She underwent Roux-en-Y gastric bypass 12 years ago. She has a history of marginal ulcers. She continues to be a smoker. Her current list of medications includes Pantoprazole, Fluoxetine, Trazodone, Pepto Bismol, Iron, Calcium, and vitamin D. Her bariatric surgeon notes blackish tongue. Which of the following statements is correct?

a. Iron deficiency is suspected.
b. The color change of tongue is likely related to her smoking
c. Bismuth sulfide is the likely reason for her black tongue
d. This condition is suggestive of acanthosis nigricans.
e. Antidepressant medications on her list are likely to cause of her black tongue.

The correct answer is "c."

Bismuth component of Pepto-Bismol combines with sulfur in saliva generating bismuth sulfide. This compound gives black colo to the tongue. It is considered harmless and stays for a brief period. Acanthosis nigricans does not involve tongue. It involves armpits, groins, skin of back of neck, and anogenital region.

Why does Pepto-Bismol sometimes darken the tongue/stool and how long does it last? (n.d.). Retrieved December 29, 2017, from http://www.pepto-bismol.com/en-us/faq/black-stool-black-tongue

**Question 34**

A 43-year-old female presents with numbness and tingling in the hands and feet. She had Roux-en-Y gastric bypass surgery 11 years ago. Her examination reveals nystagmus and some degree of confusion. Which of the following statements is correct about her clinical condition?

a. Wernicke's encephalopathy is a likely possibility
b. Absorption of thiamine is affected due to less food intake, less acid, and exclusion of duodenum
c. Concurrent B12 deficiency may also add to neural symptoms
d. Prompt treatment of the condition is needed to prevent long-term sequelae
e. All the above statements are correct

The correct answer is "e."

All the factors stated in option "b" can contribute to B1 (thiamine) deficiency. Physicians should have a high index of suspicion in dealing with any vulnerable patient. Prompt treatment can prevent long-term sequelae of Wernicke's encephalopathy. Thiamine deficiency can also lead to Beriberi. It is recognized in two forms including wet and dry types. Post gastric bypass patients with prolonged nausea and vomiting should be checked for the deficiency of B1. B12 deficiency should also be considered in patients with malabsorptive procedures.

John, Seeniann, and Carl Hoegerl. “Nutritional Deficiencies After Gastric Bypass Surgery.” The Journal of the American Osteopathic

Association, American Osteopathic Association, 1 Nov. 2009, jaoa.org/article.aspx?articleid=2093757.

## Question 35

A 33-year-old female is admitted with diarrhea and skin lesions in the form of desquamating and peeling rash at extremities and perioral areas for the last several weeks. She had Roux-en-Y gastric bypass eight years ago. She consumes alcohol on a regular basis. Her vital signs were stable. Systemic examination was otherwise normal. Her lab work showed mild anemia and mild abnormality of liver enzymes. Zinc level was 0.25 µg/mL (0.66–1.10 µg/mL). Which of the following statements is <u>not</u> correct about Zinc deficiency in Bariatric patients?

a. Zinc deficiency is suspected in the setting of post gastric bypass patients with a history of diarrhea and peeling skin rash

b. The primary absorption of zinc occurs in Jejunum

c. Niacin deficiency may have similar symptoms.

d. Most zinc deficiency cases require IV replacement of zinc.

e. Zinc sulfate, zinc gluconate, and Zinc acetate have been used for oral replacement

The correct answer is "d."

Duodenum and proximal jejunum are the primary sites for the absorption of zinc. Patients who had a duodenal switch or Roux-en-Y gastric bypass operation, are more vulnerable to zinc deficiency. Diarrhea, dermatitis, poor wound healing, cognitive dysfunction, and immune dysfunction are related clinical features. Most cases can be treated with oral zinc supplements.

Shahsavari, D., Ahmed, Z., Karikkineth, A., Williams, R., & Zigel, C. (2014). Zinc-deficiency acrodermatitis in a patient with chronic alcoholism and gastric bypass: a case report. Journal of Community Hospital Internal Medicine Perspectives, 4(3), 24707. doi:10.3402/jchimp. v4.24707

**Question 36**

A 35-year-old patient had Roux-en-Y Gastric bypass five years ago. She presents with symptoms of craving for ice and nonfood items including paper, dirt, clay, cornstarch, and paints. She feels shortness of breath on exertion. On examination, she has pallor of conjunctiva. Her health provider also notes dark circles under the eyes and spoon-shaped nails. She appears lethargic. Which of the following statements is correct about her clinical condition?

a. B12 and folic acid deficiency is suspected

b. Calcium and vitamin D deficiency is suspected.

c. Copper, Zinc deficiency is suspected

d. Iron deficiency is suspected

The correct answer is "d."

Symptoms mentioned here are suggestive of Iron deficiency. These may typically be seen in patients who had malabsorptive bariatric procedures. These include Roux-en-Y gastric bypass and duodenal switch procedures. Iron deficiency can be severe in females who have heavy periods and those who are not taking oral iron supplements regularly.

Love, A. L., & Billett, H. H. (2008). Obesity, bariatric surgery, and iron deficiency: True, true, true and related. American Journal of Hematology, 83(5), 403-409. DOI: 10.1002/ajh.21106

**Question 37**

A 32-year-old female with BMI of 48, is exploring bariatric surgery options. She is referred to a Bariatrician for a pre-operative assessment. She is interested in Roux-en-Y gastric bypass. A discussion was done about nutritional and vitamin deficiencies. The patient is especially counseled about the risks of various vitamin and micronutrient deficiencies after surgery. Which of the following statements is true regarding B12 deficiency?

a. Prevalence of B12 deficiency is not high in patients who take proton pump inhibitors

b. Serum B12 level is always adequate to identify B12 deficiency

c. Elevated Methylmalonic acid (MMA) level may be a more reliable indicator of B12 status

d. Increase serum homocysteine, and normal MMA level indicates a B12 deficiency

e. None of the above statements is true

The correct answer is "c."

Elevated Methylmalonic acid MMA has been found to be more reliable in diagnosing B12 deficiency. This test may help distinguish folic acid deficiency. Homocysteine level can be elevated in both B12 and Folic acid deficiencies.

Parrott J, Frank L, Guidelines for the Surgical Weight Loss Patient 2016 Update: Micronutrients Surg Obes Relat Dis 2017;13:727–741.

**Question 38**

A 40-year-old patient who had Roux-en-Y gastric bypass a few years ago presents to the emergency room. She had a history of recurrent marginal ulcers. Her current symptoms include persistent nausea and vomiting for the last two weeks with progressive worsening. She appears to have developed ataxia, nystagmus, confusion, and numbness. Which of the following statements is true?

a. MRI of the brain is unlikely to show increased T2 changes in thalamus, hypothalamus, enhancement of bilateral mammillary bodies and midline cerebellum

b. The deficiency is expected from a vitamin absorbed mainly in the terminal ileum

c. Her symptoms will improve with high doses of vitamin B12

d. A similar condition may be seen in chronic alcoholics

e. Her symptoms are likely to improve with high doses of vitamin D

The correct answer is "d."

Ataxia, nystagmus, and confusion with numbness can develop with B1 deficiency. This condition can be seen in alcoholics as well. Wernicke's encephalopathy needs prompt treatment with intravenous B1 administration to prevent long-term neurological sequelae. MRI scan of the brain may show changes in hypothalamus, thalamus, and related areas. In this scenario vitamin D has no role.

### Question 39

Regarding patient stated in the previous question select the correct statement

a. The patient is more likely to be a male
b. The human body has a store of the expected deficient nutrient for several months
c. Exposure of skin to sunlight help to prevent this disorder
d. Symptoms are reversible in almost all patients with adequate and timely replacement of deficient nutrient
e. As compared to a CT scan, MRI scan is more likely to hint about CNS abnormalities in this disorder

The correct answer is "e."

Condition appears to be more common in the females. Human body does not have large stores of B1. Patient with history of nausea or vomiting are more vulnerable to have B1 deficiency. Sunlight helps in production of vitamin D and not of vitamin B1. MRI scan is considered more sensitive in picking CNS abnormalities seen in Wernicke's encephalopathy.

Alias T, Hoof P, Lee M, Davis D. Wernicke's encephalopathy after conversion from sleeve gastrectomy to gastric bypass. Surgery For Obesity and Related Disease. 2016; 12:89-91

**Question 40**

Select the correct statement about recommended minimum daily intake of Vitamin D3 (Cholecalciferol) after bariatric surgery.

a. 400 international units
b. 800 international units
c. 100 international units
d. 3000 international units

The correct answer is "d."

A dose of 3000 IU to 50000 IU one to three times weekly is recommended by ASMBS, TOS and AACE.

**Question 41**

The recommended dose of daily calcium after bariatric surgery is

a. 500 mg
b. 1000 mg
c. 1200-1500 mg, and 1800-2400 mg after duodenal switch procedure.
d. 5000 mg

The correct answer is "c."

**Question 42**

Recommended daily dose of elemental Iron after bariatric surgery is

a. 10 mg
b. 45-60 mg
c. 100 mg
d. 500 mg

The correct answer is "b."

Parrott, J., Frank, L., Rabena, R., Craggs-Dino, L., Isom, K. A., & Greiman, L. (2017). American Society for Metabolic and Bariatric Surgery Integrated Health Nutritional Guidelines for the Surgical Weight Loss Patient 2016 Update: Micronutrients. Surgery for Obesity and Related Diseases, 13(5), 727-741. doi: 10.1016/j.soard.2016.12.018

**Question 43**

A female with a history of sleeve gastrectomy is seen on a follow-up visit in her primary care physician's office. Recent lab work is also available. Her hemoglobin is 9.5. Serum Iron and ferritin levels are low. She is prescribed oral iron therapy. Which of the following vitamins given concurrently can help improve iron absorption?

a. Vitamin A
b. Vitamin B2
c. Vitamin C

d. Vitamin D
e. Vitamin K

The correct answer is "c."

Vitamin C helps keep the ferric irons chelated at acid pH. It is more soluble at a high pH of the duodenum. Vitamin C is especially helpful in the absorption of iron from vegetable meals.

**Question 44**

A 42-year-old morbidly obese female with problems of DM2, HTN, and Hyperlipidemia opts for Roux-en-Y gastric bypass surgery for weight loss. Her pre-operative BMI was 52. She has a couple of C-Sections in past. Preoperative sonogram of the abdomen shows fatty liver. Gallbladder was normal. She lost about 45 pounds in four months after her bariatric procedure. She presents in the emergency with an acute right upper quadrant abdominal pain. She is currently taking medications for HTN, diabetes, oral multivitamins, and iron. She has a WBC count of 13.1, K 3.8, AST 101, ALT 92, and total bilirubin is 3.7 with a direct bilirubin level of 2.1. Please select the correct statement.

a. Rapid weight loss has no contribution to the development of her acute condition
b. Gallbladder disorder is an unlikely pathology
c. An ultrasound of right upper quadrant will be an initial investigation of choice in her case
d. Common bile duct dilates (CBD) in all cases of gastric bypass even if they do not have common bile duct stones.
e. An ERCP (endoscopic retrograde cholangiopancreatography) through the mouth can resolve her issue

The correct answer is “c."

**Question 45**

In relation to prevention and management of the problem stated in the above question, select the correct statement

a. Calcium chloride has been proven to prevent the formation of gallstones
b. Occurrence of cholesterol and bile pigment gallstones can be completely prevented with the use of bile acid products
c. Ursodeoxycholic acid is a cholesterol-lowering agent
d. Removal of the gallbladder is practiced by most surgeons to prevent gallstone complications following gastric bypass surgery
e. Patient may likely need cholecystectomy and an ERCP (endoscopic retrograde cholangiopancreatography) through the excluded stomach with operative access.

The correct answer is “e."

Gallstones and acute gallbladder condition may occur at a slightly higher frequency following rapid weight loss, especially after bariatric surgical procedures. Mobilization of cholesterol and other lipids may contribute to the development of this condition. Prophylactic removal of an otherwise normal gallbladder is not a universally accepted option. Studies have shown the reduction of gallstone incidence by approximately thirty percent with use of bile acid products following bariatric surgery. The incidence of gallstone formation is higher in initial 6 months following bariatric surgery. It has also been noted that compliance for bile acid products like ursodeoxycholic acid is poor to fair in general due to side effects. Calcium chloride may help prevent formation of renal oxalate stones. Renal stone may form at higher frequency after gastric bypass due to altered calcium and fatty acid metabolism due to malabsorption component of gastric bypass. Ultrasound is more sensitive in picking gallstones. CT scan can miss some radiolucent stones. CBD dilatation is seen in patients who have previous cholecystectomy. Up to 6mm size is considered normal. Stones in CBD can lead to common bile duct dilatation. MRI scan can be helpful to identify CBD stones.

Sattaratnamai, A., et al. "Gallstone Formation and Subsequent Cholecystectomy after Bariatric Surgery: A Systematic Review." Hpb, vol. 18, 2016, doi:10.1016/j.hpb.2016.03.375.

**Question 46**

Select the correct statement about vitamin D

a. Vitamin D is found in most naturally occurring foods
b. Vitamin D3 is produced in the skin with ultraviolet light exposure by a non-enzymatic process
c. D2 is a synthetic form (ergocalciferol)
d. All the above statements are correct.

Correct answer is "b."
Most natural foods are deficient in vitamin D. Even Milk does not contain vitamin D and is added to milk by dairy industry. Natural sunlight is a good source of vitamin D. Vitamin D3 is the form produced in skin with ultraviolet light exposure. Ability of skin to produce D3 decreases significantly beyond the age of 70. Obese patients are at higher risk of vitamin D deficiency. It can lead to secondary changes including hypocalcemia, secondary hyperparathyroidism, phosphaturia, and osteoporosis. 3000 to 6000 IU of D3 daily is recommended to treat vitamin D deficiency. 50,000 IU of D2 (ergocalciferol) one to three times a week can also be used to treat vitamin D deficiency. Ergocalciferol (D2) is found in mushrooms and other plant resources.

## Question 47

A 47-year-old female who is 5 years out from gastric bypass surgery for morbid obesity, presents with neurological symptoms affecting lower extremities. Physical examination reveals pallor of conjunctiva. She is also noted to have mild ataxia. Blood work shows anemia of microcytic type. Her hemoglobin is 9.2 and white cell count is 3700. Neutrophils are only 11%. She is in process of changing her health insurance plan and cannot afford co-pay for any additional tests. Her health care provider starts oral iron therapy with a clinical suspicion of iron deficiency. She does not take any other vitamins regularly. Patient is followed in 6 weeks. Her anemia seems not to be improving. Her symptoms of ataxia are worsened. Please select the correct statement regarding her clinical condition.

a. Her iron dose should be increased
b. She should continue with Iron with a B12 shot in the office
c. Selenium deficiency should be suspected
d. Zinc deficiency may be the reason for her symptoms
e. Copper deficiency should be suspected

Correct answer is "e."

Copper deficiency could be a reason. Copper level should be checked in her case. Copper is absorbed in stomach and duodenum. Patients with a history of gastric bypass surgery are vulnerable to copper deficiency. Copper deficiency in malabsorptive procedures like Roux-en-Y gastric bypass and duodenal switch operations is rare but a well-documented condition.

**Question 48**

A patient with history of gastric bypass 12 years ago is diagnosed with copper deficiency. She takes iron for anemia and low ferritin levels. She has received iron infusions in the past. She takes Zinc regularly as well for low Zinc levels. Medical reconciliation reveals that she takes a multivitamin preparation containing molybdenum and selenium. She is advised to take copper sulphate preparation for the copper deficiency. Which of the following supplements can conflict with the absorption of copper?

a. Iron
b. Zinc
c. Selenium
d. Molybdenum

Correct answer is "b."

Zinc and Copper compete for absorption. Concurrent ingestion of Zinc for a long period of time can lead to copper deficiency. This can result in myelopathy.

https://www.uptodate.com/contents/copper-deficiency-myeloneuropathy?search=copper%20deficiency&source=search_result&selectedTitle=1~60&usage_type=default&display_rank=1

## Question 49

A post gastric bypass patient who is currently a smoker presents with pain in epigastric area. She smokes a pack daily. She has developed marginal ulcers in the past and had one incidence of marginal ulcer perforation requiring laparoscopic repair. An attempt to quit smoking in past caused her to gain weight. Bariatric surgeon is working closely with family physician to help her stop smoking. A decision is made to check her biochemistry randomly for compliance for nonsmoking. Please select the correct statement.

a. Nicotine half-life is about 0.5 to 3 hours and for Continine it is about 16 to 19 hours
b. Tobacco cigarette and "vaping" e-cigarettes produce similar level of continine
c. Gastric bypass status does not alter the pharmacokinetics or dynamics of nicotine
d. Stopping smoking frequently results in weight gain
e. All above statements are correct

Correct answer is "e."

Statements (a) to (d) are correct. Continine level is the preferred test to check for tobacco use and compliance for nonsmoking. Some of the other short-lived metabolites useful to check for smoking status include anabasine and nornicotine. Nicotine does carry a suppressant effect on appetite. Smoking increases the risk of developing and non-healing of marginal ulcers.

## Question 50

A 19-year-old girl is diagnosed with polycystic ovaries. She has a BMI of 39. She has irregular periods. Lab work shows high insulin levels suggestive of insulin resistance. She is started on metformin. She also sees a nutritionist and a counselor. She is told about the possibility of use of this medication on long-term basis. She will be prone to have which of the following deficiencies with long-term use of metformin.?

a. Vitamin B1

b. Vitamin B2

c. Vitamin B6

d. Vitamin B12

e. None of the above vitamin deficiency is associated with long-term use of metformin

The correct answer is "d."

Pediatric Obesity—Assessment, Treatment, and Prevention ... academic.oup.com/jcem/article/102/3/709/2965084.

## Question 51

A 16-year-old girl is started on prescription strength Orlistat to help lose weight. She is also diagnosed with hypothyroidism and takes levothyroxine. She lost 12 pounds in the last 4 months. Her family is very supportive. She has made dietary changes and goes to gym regularly. She presents in the emergency department with severe right upper quadrant pain. Please select to correct statement.

a. Liver functions need to be monitored
b. Biliary stones can form with the use of orlistat
c. Levothyroxine level may drop with use of orlistat
d. Renal function impairment may happen
e. All the above statements are correct

The correct answer is "e."

All the statements from "a" to "d" are correct.

Pediatric Obesity—Assessment, Treatment, and Prevention ... academic.oup.com/jcem/article/102/3/709/2965084.

**Question 52**

A 19-year-old girl is found to have insulin resistance. Her BMI is 43. Her insulin level is in range of 35 to 40. She is started on metformin 500 mg orally twice daily. After two day she calls the office complaining of abdominal pain and diarrhea. Please select to correct statement about her condition.

a. Switching to slow-release preparation of metformin may <u>not</u> be helpful
b. Clostridium Difficile infections are common after metformin use
c. Metformin causes bowel ischemia leading to diarrhea and pain
d. Genetic variation may exist regarding side effects and tolerance for metformin

Correct answer is “d.”

Slow-release preparation may be better tolerated in some patients. C Diff infections have closer association with use of antibiotics. Metformin does not cause bowel ischemia. Genetic variations in metformin intolerance exist and this is an area of interest in research.

McCreight, Laura J et al. “Metformin and the gastrointestinal tract.” *Diabetologia* vol. 59,3 (2016): 426-35. doi:10.1007/s00125-015-3844-9

**Question 53**

The common nutritional deficiencies seen in obstetric patients after Roux- en-Y gastric bypass surgery include all the following EXCEPT.

a. Vitamin C

b. Iron

c. Folate

d. Vitamin D

e. Vitamin B12

The correct answer is “a.”

The common nutritional deficiencies after Roux-en-Y gastric bypass surgery are of protein, iron, vitamin B12, folate, vitamin D, and calcium.

It is important to recognize specific dietary and micronutrient needs of pregnant women who have undergone Roux-en-Y gastric bypass surgery. Vitamin A needs to be in the form of beta-carotene. 5000 IU is the recommended dose. Vitamin A has teratogenic effects. B12 should be given in a dose of 1mg intramuscular every third month. Thiamine recommendations include 50mg daily. Dose may need to be increased in patient with poor intake with excessive nausea or vomiting. Such patients carry risk of developing Wernicke's encephalopathy. Folic acid recommendation is 400 mcg in first 12 weeks and 5mg in later weeks.

High risk of deficiencies demand monitoring of labs in each trimester.

ACOG Practice Bulletin No. 105: Bariatric Surgery and...: Obstetrics & Gynecology. (n.d.). Retrieved January 06, 2018, from http://journals.lww.com/greenjournal/Citation/2009/06000/ACOG_Practice_Bulletin_No__105__Bariatric_Surgery.48.aspx

**Question 54**

A morbidly obese 30-year-old female is referred to her OB/GYN physician for counseling about appropriate birth control options. She is on a combination oral contraceptive pill regimen. She is also following with a bariatric practice. She is using Topiramate phentermine combination for the last couple of months for weight loss. Which of the following statements is correct?

a. The patient may experience breakthrough bleeding

b. Ethinyl estradiol levels may become lower by 30% with concurrent topiramate use

c. Ethinyl estradiol levels may become higher by 30% with concurrent topiramate use

d. Ethinyl estradiol levels are not changed with concurrent topiramate use

e. Norethindrone levels are increased by 50% with concurrent topiramate use

f. a and b are correct

The correct answer is "f."

It has been observed that levels of estrogen component of oral contraceptive pills may become lower with concurrent use of topiramate. This can result in breakthrough bleedings.

Rosenfeld, W. E., Doose, D. R., Walker, S. A., & Nayak, R. K. (1997). Effect of Topiramate on the Pharmacokinetics of an Oral Contraceptive Containing Norethindrone and Ethinyl Estradiol in Patients with Epilepsy. Epilepsia, 38(3), 317-323. doi:10.1111/j.1528-1157.1997.tb01123.x

**Question 55**

A 24-year-old female patient who is gravida 0 presents with complaints of oligomenorrhea, excessive facial hair and weight gain. Physical exam shows BMI 41, hirsutism, acanthosis nigricans, abdominal striae with pannus, and Tanner's stage IV development. Patient's workup shows negative urine pregnancy test, elevated HbA1C, elevated fasting blood sugar, deranged lipid profile, elevated fasting serum insulin, elevated free testosterone, normal DHEAS, normal 17 hydroxyprogesterone acetate, normal TSH and normal prolactin. 24-hour urinary free cortisol excretion test is normal. Which of the following differential diagnoses is suspected?

a. Adrenal hyperplasia

b. PCOS (polycystic ovarian syndrome)
c. Cushing's syndrome
d. Hypothyroidism
e. Hyperprolactinemia

The correct answer is "b."

**Question 56**

What would be the next management steps in the case discussed above?

a. Pelvic ultrasound
b. Progesterone challenge followed by combined birth control pills
c. Metformin
d. Counseling about weight loss and healthy lifestyle
e. All the above statements are correct

The correct answer is "e."

**Question 57**

A 23-year-old female is seeing her family physician for annual physical. She is thinking to start oral contraceptives for birth control. She has concerns about weight gain with the use of this type of contraception. Please select the correct statement.

a. Current oral contraceptives have a great potential to cause weight gain due to estrogen content
b. Fat storage is more likely than fluid retention to cause weight gain with use of oral contraceptives
c. Older contraceptives had high estrogen content, and these were more likely to cause weight gain.
d. Progesterone component of oral contraceptives is a likely factor in causing weight gain

The correct answer is "c."

Older oral contraceptives which were available several decades ago, had high estrogen levels. These led to weight gain by increasing hunger and fluid retention, in many women. Current generation of oral contraceptives have low estrogens. These are not thought to cause significant weight gain. Any patient using these medications should be aware of these facts. Dietary counseling may help in the patients prone to gain weight.

**Question 58**

Please select the correct statement regarding interaction of naltrexone bupropion (Contrave ®) combination with other medicines.

a. No need of adjusting dose while taking clopidogrel
b. Clopidogrel dose need to be increased while taking naltrexone bupropion combination
c. Clopidogrel interaction with naltrexone/bupropion combination occurs due to inhibition of cytochrome CYP2B6 by the former.
d. Dextromethorphan containing cough suppressant can be used safely with naltrexone/bupropion combination

The correct answer is "c."

Clopidogrel inhibits cytochrome CYP2B6. This will impair the metabolism of the naltrexone/bupropion combination. This requires the dose of this combination to be reduced. Anti-opioid component "naltrexone" will render opioids ineffective if used concurrently.
https://contravehcp.com/dosing/

**Question 59**

A patient is taking bupropion for reasons of depression. She is not taking any other medications currently. Her BMI is 34. She is interested in trying phentermine to help lose weight. Her family physician discusses the potential risks and benefits of using phentermine and bupropion together. Select the correct statement.

a. Risk of seizures will be increased
b. Two medicines can be used safely. No interaction is expected
c. Risk of arrhythmias increases
d. Dose of phentermine needs to be increased
e. Effect of phentermine will be blunted if used together with bupropion

The correct answer is "a."
Risk of seizures may increase with concurrent use of phentermine and bupropion.
https://www.drugs.com/drug-interactions/phentermine-with-wellbutrin-1851-0-440-203.html#:~:text=buPROPion%20phentermine&text=BuPROPion%20may%20rarely%20cause%20seizures,phentermine%20may%20increase%20that%20risk.

**Question 60**

Phentermine and bupropion combined use risk related to seizures increases in which of the following circumstances?

a. Elderly age group
b. History of brain trauma
c. Alcohol or drug withdrawal
d. Presence of brain tumor
e. All above are correct

The correct answer is "e."
All the choices are correct.
https://www.drugs.com/drug-interactions/phentermine-with-wellbutrin-1851-0-440-203.html#:~:text=buPROPion%20phentermine&text=BuPROPion%20may%20rarely%20cause%20seizures,phentermine%20may%20increase%20that%20risk.

**Question 61**

Which of the following anesthetic has shown to reduce post operative use of narcotics and better pain control in Bariatric patients?

a. Dexmedetomidine (DEX)
b. Nitrous oxide
c. Halothane
d. isoflurane

The correct answer is "a."
Dexmedetomidine belongs to alpha-2 adrenergic receptor agonist family. It produces its beneficial effect probably by reducing the surge of catecholamines and reduced need of volatile anesthetics and opioid agents.
Jin S, Liang DD, Chen C, Zhang M, Wang J. Dexmedetomidine prevent postoperative nausea and vomiting on patients during general anesthesia: A PRISMA-compliant meta-analysis of

randomized controlled trials. Medicine (Baltimore). 2017;96(1):e5770. doi:10.1097/MD.0000000000005770

## Question 62

Thrombotic events after bariatric surgery remain a concerning issue. Better evaluation can help decide about extended DVT prophylaxis. Studies have included panels focusing on factor VIII, protein C, protein S, antithrombin III, and activated protein C resistance. Please select the correct statement

a. Factor VIII elevation is most common anomaly
b. Factor VIII deficiency is most common anomaly
c. Protein C and S deficiency is most common anomaly
d. Protein C resistance is most common anomaly

The correct answer is “a.”
Thrombophilia is prevalent in in more than 50% patients seeking sleeve gastrectomy procedure. Factor VIII elevation is found to be the most common anomaly. Extended chemoprophylaxis may decrease portal vein thrombosis risk.
https://link.springer.com/article/10.1007/s11695-009-9906-7

## Question 63

In bariatric practice a term “carbohydrate loading” is used. Please select the statement which describes this term correctly?

a. It is the bulk of carbohydrate taken before a ketogenic diet protocol is started
b. It is the parenteral carbohydrate load given once nutritional rehabilitation started for a severely malnourished case after any malabsorptive procedure
c. It is the carbohydrate containing drink given on the day of bariatric surgery a couple of hours before anesthesia for various benefits
d. It refers to the carbohydrate load ingested in very low-calorie diet protocols.

The correct answer is "c."
Carbohydrate loading refers to carbohydrate containing drink about 2 hours before the procedure. This helps to reduce insulin resistance, decreases protein loss, and decrease hospital stay. It is shown not affect gastric emptying adversely.
Kratzing C. Pre-operative nutrition and carbohydrate loading. Proc Nutr Soc. 2011 Aug;70(3):311-5. doi: 10.1017/S0029665111000450. PMID: 21781358.

**Question 64**

Thromboembolic complications after bariatric surgery have always been a big concern. Pulmonary embolism is one of the most common causes of mortality after bariatric surgery. Different dosing regimens are used to achieve therapeutic effect with enoxaparin in post operative period. It is estimated that about 15% of morbidly obese patients remain subtherapeutic once given enoxaparin. There are concerns of overdosing as well. Which of the following can be used to determine the adequacy of prophylaxis?

a. Anti-factor Xa
b. Anti-factor XI
c. Anti-factor VII
d. Anti-factor V

The correct answer is "a."
Anti-factor Xa can be used to a assess the adequacy of thromboprophylaxis. It is checked generally 3 to 5 hours after the second dose of enoxaparin.

Assessment of empiric body mass index-based thromboprophylaxis dosing of enoxaparin after bariatric surgery: evidence for dosage adjustment using anti-factor Xa in high-risk patients
Linden A. Karas, M.D. Zubaidah Nor Hanipah, M.D. Derrik Cetin D.O. et al

## Question 65

A pharmacy service contacts the physician regarding a patient's medication profile. Patient is post gastric sleeve surgery 3 years ago. The note from the pharmacy raises concerns about pantoprazole sodium. Patients insurance claim records also reveal presence of anemia. Please select the correct statement.

a. Iron deficiency could be contributing to the anemia
b. B12 deficiency could be contributing to the anemia
c. PPI related hypochlorhydria can impair the absorption of iron
d. More intensive iron therapy may be necessary
e. All the above statements are correct

The correct answer is "e."
All the statements are correct. Use of PPI can lead to hypochlorhydria leading to iron and B12 malabsorption.

## Question 66

A patient with sleeve gastrectomy is suffering from severe symptoms of GERD. He is started on Pantoprazole sodium once daily. Symptoms fail to improve. Dose of pantoprazole is adjusted and now he takes BID dose. Symptoms get controlled. Patient stays on this regimen for more than a year. Pharmacy sends a letter to the prescribing physician with concerns regarding high dose of PPI for long duration. Letter mentions some nutritional deficiency risks. High dose and chronic use of pantoprazole may result in deficiency of which of the following

a. Potassium
b. Magnesium
c. sodium
d. zinc
e. All the above statements are correct

The correct answer is "b."

Chronic high dose use of pantoprazole may result in hypomagnesemia.

**Question 67**

Bariatric surgery can affect thyroid status. Which of the following may be expected after significant weight loss?

a. Resolution of subclinical hypothyroidism, decreased TSH level, decreased levothyroxine dose
b. Resolution of subclinical hypothyroidism, increased TSH level, and increased levothyroxine dose
c. No effect on hypothyroidism, TSH level unchanged and decreased dose of levothyroxine
d. Worsening of subclinical hypothyroidism, increased TSH level and no change of levothyroxine dose
e. All the above statements are correct

The correct answer is "a."
A recently published metanalysis determines that bariatric surgery has association with resolution of subclinical hypothyroidism, decreased TSH levels and need of decreased dose of levothyroxine.

Hypothyroidism and levothyroxine therapy following bariatric surgery: a systematic review, meta-analysis, network metanalysis, and meta- regression CArmil Azran,Pham.D., Nirvana Hanhan-Shamshoum, Tujan Irshied Soard Voume 17, Issue 6 P1206-1217

**Question 68**

Clinical practice guidelines recommend

a. Avoid using extended-release ER formulations in post bariatric surgery situations
b. Absorption surface area is increased for extended-release formulations in a gastric bypass patient due to rerouting o bowel
c. Intermediate-release (IR) and non-absorbable sugar containing liquid formulations are not preferred in post bariatric surgery patients.
d. Efficacy of extended-release medications is increased afte gastric bypass surgery
e. All the above statements are correct

The correct answer is "a."
Based upon a recent study it appears that extended-release preparations should be avoided in post bariatric patients. This study looked at the data related gastric bypass and sleeve gastrectomy patients. Potential untoward effects are attributed to the use of extended-release formulations in this category of the patients.
Changes in utilization of immediate-release, extended-release, and liquid formulation medications relative to bariatric surgery: a segmented regression analysis Scott Martin Vouri 1, Hemita Bhagwandass 2, et all Obes Relat Dis. Surg 2021 Jun;17(6):1089-1094. doi: 10.1016/j.soard.2021.02.027. Epub 2021 Mar 3.

**Question 69**

Morbidly obese patients are vulnerable to have thiamine deficiency. Please select the correct statement.

a. Females with shorter height are likely to have higher thiamine levels
b. Taller males are likely to have higher thiamine levels

c. Human body have stores of thiamine which can be sufficient for many months
d. Adipose tissues are rich in thiamine
e. All the above statements are correct

The correct answer is “b.”

Human body has limited thiamine stores. Skeletal muscles have higher concentration of thiamine. Taller males with more muscular mass are likely to have higher thiamine levels. Obese patients in perioperative period are more vulnerable to thiamine deficiency. This can have serious neurological consequences including Korsakoff psychosis or Wernicke encephalopathy.

Prevalence of thiamine deficiency is significant in patients undergoing primary bariatric surgery

VAncel. Albaugh, M.D., Brandon Williams, M.D. et all

**Question 70**

Vitamin E plays role in several body processes. Please select the correct statement.

a. Vitamin E is a fat-soluble vitamin
b. Vitamin E deficiency is some time seen in post bariatric surgery patients
c. Patients with malabsorption type bariatric procedures are affected more
d. Vitamin E is stored predominantly in adipose tissues
e. Neuropathy, myopathy, gait disturbances, sensory loss, ataxia, immune disorders, and ophthalmologic deficits are some of the clinical manifestations of the deficiency
f. All the above are correct

The correct answer is “f.”

Vitamin E is a one of the fat-soluble vitamins. It is found in plants. Seeds, nuts, green leafy vegetables, vegetable oils and fish naturally contain this vitamin. In human body its benefits include antioxidant properties, immune effects, modulation of enzymes and signal transduction. This vitamin is mainly absorbed in proximal bowel. Dose recommendations are not well defined at present.
Vitamin E status among bariatric surgery patients: a systematic review
Shiri Sherf-Degn, R.D., PhD, Assaf Buch R.D., Ph.D, et all

**Question 71**

Please select the correct statement regarding use of vitamins in pregnant patients

a. Retinoids are not safe to use during pregnancy
b. Beta carotenes can be used in pregnancy
c. B12 and folic acid are teratogenic
d. Options "a." and "b." are correct
e. All the above statements are correct

The correct answer is "d."

**Question 72**

Dexmedetomidine has been in focus in Bariatric surgery. What is the pharmacological importance of this medication?

a. It is a betablocker. It helps control heart rate
b. It is a highly selective alpha-2 adrenergic receptor agonist. It is found useful in post operative nausea control
c. It is a weight loss medication
d. It helps control Binge eating

The correct answer is "b."

**Question 73**

Select the correct statement regarding Dexmedetomidine therapeutic effects.

a. Sedation
b. Analgesia
c. Anxiolytic
d. Less respiratory depression
e. All above statements are correct

The correct answer is "e."
Dexmedetomidine has gained interest regarding prevention of postoperative nausea after bariatric surgery. A lot of emphasis is being made recently to cut down use of narcotics in bariatric surgery practice. " BStop" initiative is one the quality improvement projects by the leading organizations in the field. This medicine is found beneficial regarding reducing the dose of opioids in the perioperative period. It is also shown to cause appreciable reduction in postoperative pain scores.
Editorial Comment on: Postoperative nausea and vomiting after bariatric surgery and dexmedetomidine anesthetic: a propensity-weighted analysis. Surgery for Obesity and Related Disease 16 (2020) e39-e40

**Question 74**

Iron absorption can be altered in certain situations. Please select the correct statement regarding oral iron therapy.

a. Absorption of iron can be impaired if calcium and iron are taken at the same time
b. Absorption of iron is enhanced if it is taken along with calcium
c. Absorption of iron is decreased if vitamin C is taken concurrently
d. All the above statements are correct

The correct answer is "a."

Iron absorption can be impaired if it is taken along with calcium. Timing of intake of calcium and iron should be at least 2 hours apart. Low calcium content is seen in some dedicated bariatric vitamin preparations for the same reasons.

**Question 75**

Please select the correct statement about use of specialized vitamins after bariatric surgery.

a. It is not important to take specialized vitamins after bariatric surgery
b. Taking specialized vitamins is more important in prevention of various deficiencies in sleeve gastrectomy patients only.
c. Taking specialized vitamins is more important in prevention of various deficiencies in gastric bypass patients
d. Taking specialized vitamins is more important in prevention of various deficiencies in gastric adjustable band patients.

The correct answer is "c."
Gastric bypass patient may see deficiencies more often related to iron, B12, folic acid, and vitamin D. Malabsorption and small stomach size contributes various nutritional deficiencies.
Do specialized bariatric multivitamins lower deficiencies after RYGB
Wendy Schijns, MD, Lisanne T. Schuurman, MD, Alida Melse-Boonstra, MD et al Surgery for Obesity and Related Disease 14(2018) 1005-1002

## Question 76

Warfarin management in perioperative period in bariatric patients poses several challenges. Please select the correct statement.

a. Warfarin is mainly absorbed in terminal ileum, so its dose and levels are not affected by a Roux-en-Y gastric bypass.
b. It is observed that in gastric bypass patients dose requirements tend to be lower in first month and later increase
c. Warfarin is mainly metabolized in renal tissues
d. Warfarin dose requires to be increased in immediate post operative period as most absorption of warfarin occurs in proximal duodenum.

The correct answer is "b."
Warfarin is mainly absorbed in proximal duodenum however due to various other factors not completely understood, the dose requirements remain lower in immediate postoperative period after gastric bypass. A dose reduction by approximately 25% or more may be required in early post operative period. Warfarin is metabolized in liver by enzymes CYP2C9 and CYP3A4 of cytochrome p450 group.

Andew T. Strong, MD, Guatam Sharma et al SOARD VOLUME 14 ISSUE 5 P700-706 MAY 01 2018

https://doi.org/10.1016/j.soard.2017.12021

## Question 77

Which of the following medications have shown some benefit in Obese patients with diabetes and non-alcoholic fatty liver disease?

a. Metformin.
b. Liraglutide
c. Sitagliptin

d. Pioglitazone

The correct answer is “d.”
Pioglitazone has shown some improvement in numbers regarding haptic fat content. No improvement is noted in fibrosis scores. Patient on pioglitazone can have some weight gain.

Blazina, I., Selph, S. Diabetes drugs for nonalcoholic fatty liver disease: a systematic review. Syst Rev 8, 295 (2019). https://doi.org/10.1186/s13643-019-1200-8

**Question 78**

A patient who is following a weight loss program calls to have an appointment to discuss trying semaglutide. She read about this medicine on internet. Please select the correct statement.

a. This a GLP1 agonist
b. It is once a week injectable preparation for weight loss.
c. It cannot be used in patients with history of medullary thyroid cancer or Type 2 multiple endocrine neoplasia syndrome
d. Some of the side effects include, pancreatitis, gallstones, renal impairment, risk of hypoglycemia, depression, and suicidal ideations
e. All the above statements are correct

correct answer is “e.”
Semaglutide (Wegovy ™) * is a glucagon-like peptide-1 (GLP-1) agonist. This injectable medication increases secretion of insulin. It is given once a week and dose is titrated to a higher level with monthly increments. An oral version of this medicine is available to treat diabetes.

https://en.wikipedia.org/wiki/Semaglutide#cite_note-FDA2019-18

https://www.wegovy.com/?gclid=Cj0KCQjwnoqLBhD4ARIsAL5JedJCUJgSctJNitfXT2Tljmaxq7J_oeZ65M-YUZE1pxjPDgUUmSuWDQEaArVQEALw_wcB&gclsrc=aw.ds

* Wegovy™ is a trademark of Novo Nordisk A/S.

**Question 79**

Please select the correct statement about semaglutide?

a. Dose adjustment is needed in patients with renal impairment
b. Dose adjustment is needed in patients with hepatic impairment
c. Dose adjustment is needed in patients with both renal and hepatic impairments
d. Dose adjustment is not needed in patients with both renal and hepatic impairments

The correct answer is "d."
Semaglutide (Wegovy ™) clinical trial has shown no clinically relevant change in patients with both renal and hepatic impairments. However, it should be kept in mind that symptoms related to nausea, vomiting and diarrhea can lead to acute renal injury especially in patients with preexisting renal impairment. In clinical trials it has been used in patients above 65 years of age. Safety and efficacy were comparable to younger patients
https://www.novo-pi.com/wegovy.pdf

**Question 80**

Semaglutide should be discontinued before planned pregnancy. It is suggested that the drug should be discontinued at least how much time before?

a. 5 days
b. 10 days
c. 2 weeks
d. 4 weeks
e. 2 months

The correct answer is “e.”
Semaglutide has a long half-life of 1 week. Drug may be present in the body system 4 to 7 weeks following a dose of 2.4 mg. Extensive binding to plasma protein slows its degradation and clearance through the kidneys.
https://www.novo-pi.com/wegovy.pdf

**Question 81**

Please select the correct statement about Semaglutide

a. Its action through GLP 1 receptors include reduction of insulin production
b. Its action through GLP 1 receptors include increased production of insulin
c. Its action through GLP 1 receptors include reduction of glucagon production
d. Its action through GLP 1 receptors include increased production of glucagon
e. Options (b) and (c) are correct

The correct answer is “e.”
Semaglutide (Wegovy ™) causes increased production of insulin and decreases production of glucagon. These effects help in lowering blood sugar.
https://www.novo-pi.com/wegovy.pdf

**Question 82**

Semaglutide is GLP1 analogue, and it acts through GLP 1 receptor

a. Semaglutide acts through its action on GLP 1 receptors present in pancreas
b. Semaglutide acts through its action on GLP 1 receptors present in Liver

c. Semaglutide acts through its action on GLP 1 receptors present in fat cells
d. Semaglutide acts through its action on GLP 1 receptors present in brain
e. Options (a) and (b) are correct

The correct answer is "d."
Semaglutide acts through its action on appetite control centers in brain by its action on GLP1 receptors.
https://www.novo-pi.com/wegovy.pdf

**Question 83**

Please select the correct statement about ICG (indocyanine green dye) use in management of obese patients

a. Can be used to assess fatty liver
b. Can help visualize biliary ductal structures during bariatric surgery and concurrent cholecystectomy
c. Can help assess vascularity of tissues during bariatric surgical procedures
d. Can help assess anastomosis integrity by injecting in the stomach
e. All the above statements are correct

The correct answer is "e."
ICG dye is used very commonly in surgical practices. It produces fluorescent green color. This can be picked with special cameras during laparoscopic / robotic and other procedures. This property makes it useful to identify vascularity of tissues in addition to the uses mentioned above.
Carrano, F. M., & Di Lorenzo, N. (2020). The use of indocyanine green in bariatric surgery: A systematic review. Journal of Gastric Surgery, 2(2), 41–44. https://doi.org/10.36159/jgs.v2i2.47

## Question 84

Which of the following chemotherapeutic agents should be given according to predicted normal weight of an obese patient?

a. Paclitaxel
b. Troxacitabine
c. Irinotecan
d. Cicplatin
e. Carboplatin

The correct answer is "e."
Doses of options (a) to (d) should be calculated according to surface area. However, carboplatin should be dosed according to predicted normal weight of the patient.
https://journals.lww.com/oncology-times/fulltext/2012/02250/how_obesity_complicates_cancer_treatment.1.aspx

## Question 85

Tendencies among oncologists exist to reduce the doses of various chemotherapeutic agents to lessen risks of toxicity in obese patients. Please select the correct statement about American society of clinical oncology guidelines regarding dosing issue.

a. Panel suggest full weight-based dosing of cytotoxic chemotherapeutic agents
b. Full approved doses of immune and targeted therapies in obese adults cancer patients
c. In case of toxicity doses should be modified and handled similarly in nonobese and obese patients
d. Fixed dose therapy is limited to select cytotoxic agents like bleomycin
e. All above statements are correct

The correct answer is “e.”
Guidelines published in 2021 state the above facts.

DOI: 10.1200/JCO.21.00471 Journal of Clinical Oncology 39, no. 18 (June 20, 2021) 2037-2048.

**Question 86**

There is limited data about dosing guidelines for many commonly used medications in critically sick obese patients. Which of the following medications is recommended to have standard dose without size descriptor?

a. Non opioid analgesics
b. ketamine
c. Opioid analgesics
d. None of the above medications is recommended to have dosing without size descriptor

The correct answer is “a.”
Non opioids are recommended to be used with standard doses.
For Ketamine and opioids, ideal or adjusted body weight should be used to calculate doses.
Erstad, B.L., Barletta, J.F. Drug dosing in the critically ill obese patient—a focus on sedation, analgesia, and delirium. Crit Care 24, 315 (2020). https://doi.org/10.1186/s13054-020-03040-z

**Question 87**

Which of the following sedative medications are recommended to be used according to actual body weight when BMI is less than 40 $kg/m^2$?

a. Propofol
b. Midazolam

c. Dexmedetomidine
d. Etomidate

The correct answer is "d."
Etomidate is recommended to be used with actual body weight when BMI is less than 40 and for BMI more than 40 adjusted or actual body weight should be used. For propofol, Dexmedetomidine and Midazolam ideal or adjusted body weight should be used. Similarly ideal weight should be used for midazolam while giving infusions.
Erstad, B.L., Barletta, J.F. Drug dosing in the critically ill obese patient—a focus on sedation, analgesia, and delirium. Crit Care 24, 315 (2020). https://doi.org/10.1186/s13054-020-03040-z

**Question 88**

Which of the following medications can be used with standard, non-weight-based doses in obese critically sick patients?

a. Propofol
b. Quetiapine
c. Dexmedetomidine
d. Haloperidol
e. Options (b) and (d) are correct

The correct answer is "d."
Quetiapine and haloperidol are used with standard, non-weigh-based doses.
Erstad, B.L., Barletta, J.F. Drug dosing in the critically ill obese patient—a focus on sedation, analgesia, and delirium. Crit Care 24, 315 (2020). https://doi.org/10.1186/s13054-020-03040-z

**Question 89**

A 55-year-old female who is post Roux-en-Y gastric bypass develops internal hernia with strangulation. Major small bowel resection was done. After a long hospital stay, she is discharged to a rehab facility with total parenteral nutritional support. She is counseled about her future options to manage short bowel syndrome. Which of the following medications can potentially help her?

a. GLP-1 agonist
b. Leptin injections
c. GLP-2 agonist
d. Insulin injections

Correct answer is "c."

Teduglutide (brand name Gattex) is a GLP-2 agonist. It promotes mucosal growth, gastric emptying, and stomach secretions. Development of tumors, hepatobiliary disease, fluid overload, intestinal obstruction and altered absorption of some of the drugs are few of the side effects. Potential for various malignancies is a concerning issue. Leptin and insulin have no specific role in short bowel syndrome management. GLP 1 agonists have been used in treatment of diabetes and lately also for weight loss.

Notes

Notes

https://www.facebook.com/MedicalFronts

**Subscribe to Newsletter**

https://medicalfronts.com/index.php/subscribe-to-newsletter/

**Learn about additional study resources**

**OBESITY MULTIPLE CHOICE QUESTIONS 4th EDITION 2022**

**(Available at Amazon)**

**THE OBESITY: Multiple Choice Questions Learn & Prepare (Book)**

**and**

**Obesity Insights and Learning: Self-Assessment Exam**

*(Another resource to practice obesity related questions)*

https://medicalfronts.com/index.php/obesity-insights-and-learning/

Made in United States
Orlando, FL
07 June 2026

82451103R10044